Aline Beatriz Rocha Paula
Francisco B. M. Oliveira

Temporomandibular Dysfunction, Lipodystrophy Syndrome and Depression

AF303508

Aline Beatriz Rocha Paula
Francisco B. M. Oliveira

Temporomandibular Dysfunction, Lipodystrophy Syndrome and Depression

A risk assessment of people living with HIV/AIDS

ScienciaScripts

Imprint
Any brand names and product names mentioned in this book are subject to trademark, brand or patent protection and are trademarks or registered trademarks of their respective holders. The use of brand names, product names, common names, trade names, product descriptions etc. even without a particular marking in this work is in no way to be construed to mean that such names may be regarded as unrestricted in respect of trademark and brand protection legislation and could thus be used by anyone.

Cover image: www.ingimage.com

This book is a translation from the original published under ISBN 978-613-9-62918-3.

Publisher:
Sciencia Scripts
is a trademark of
Dodo Books Indian Ocean Ltd. and OmniScriptum S.R.L publishing group

120 High Road, East Finchley, London, N2 9ED, United Kingdom
Str. Armeneasca 28/1, office 1, Chisinau MD-2012, Republic of Moldova, Europe
Printed at: see last page
ISBN: 978-620-7-75713-8

SUMMARY

ACKNOWLEDGMENTS

I would first like to thank God for blessing me and helping me get this far, for putting people in my path who have helped me along the way.

To my parents, Natanael Paula and Gilvana Rocha, for their lessons, advice and all the support I needed throughout this journey, even though words cannot express my gratitude to you.

To all my friends, for their experiences, encouragement and companionship throughout this time.

To my advisor, Francisco Braz Milanez Oliveira, for his patience, for demanding more of me so that I could excel, for the criticism and praise that only contributed to my growth, for his professionalism, helpfulness and availability.

My professors Dr. Ana Carla Marques da Costa, Ms. Màrcia Sousa Santos and Ms. Ana Elizabeth Félix for helping me when I needed it. And to all the teachers, masters and doctors, who contributed to my learning during my academic journey.

I dedicate this work to my parents Natanael Paula and Gilvana Rocha, my brother Eduardo, my friends and teachers for their dedication, love, support, encouragement and trust during this stage in my life.

1. INTRODUCTION

Temporomandibular dysfunction (TMD) is the general term used to explain the various clinical conditions that affect the masticatory muscles, the temporomandibular joint and associated structures (CALIXTRE et al., 2014; ZAVANELLI et al., 2013; MACHADO et al., 2010).

The main signs and symptoms of TMD are: orofacial pain, joint noise, limited range of jaw movements, headache, otalgia, ear fullness, hearing loss, tinnitus, vertigo, painful palpation of temporomandibular structures, sleep disorders, asymptomatic radiographic changes, including pain, bruxism, depression and stress (CAMACHO et al., 2014; DALL' ANTONIA et al., 2013; LEITE et al., 2013; ORTEGA; GUIMARÂES, 2013; PIZOLATO; FERNANDES; GAVIÂO, 2013; SENA et al., 2013; ZAVANELLI et al., 2013; PASINATO et al., 2011; MACHADO et al., 2010; DONNARUMMA et al., 2010; MORENO et al., 2009; SANTOS et al., 2006).

From the available literature, it can be seen that the etiology of TMD can be proven to stem from behavioral and environmental patterns, regardless of the individual's genetics, and are amenable to intervention (ORTEGA; GUIMARÂES, 2013). Thus, diagnosis and multi-professional treatment are two important parts of effective treatment (ZAVANELLI et al., 2013; BONJARDIM et al., 2005).

Some variables such as gender and age influence the clinical expression of TMD, affecting adults more frequently, especially females; however, signs and symptoms of TMD have been observed in children and the elderly (SENA et al., 2013; CAMACHO et al., 2014; MAZZETTO et al., 2014).

It can therefore be inferred that people living with the Human Immunodeficiency Virus (HIV) or Acquired Immunodeficiency Syndrome (AIDS) (PLWHA) are also exposed to these risk factors, considering that TMD affects the general population.

The lipodystrophic syndrome is an adverse effect of the antiretroviral therapy (ART) used by HIV/AIDS patients: hypertriglyceridemia, hypercholesterolemia and other metabolic alterations such as insulin resistance, hyperglycemia and redistribution of body fat (lipodystrophy), leading to increased arterial stiffness and the incidence of myocardial infarction, The combination of these changes is known as Human Immunodeficiency Virus Lipodystrophy Syndrome (HIV-LS), in addition to difficulties in social and sexual relationships, loss of self-esteem and social isolation (ARMENTANO et al., 2013; SOARES; COSTA, 2013; DOMINGOS et al., 2012; EIRA et al., 2012; GODOI et al., 2012; ROMANCINI et al., 2012; ANJOS et al., 2011; CECCATO et al., 2011; SEGATTO et al., 2011; DUTRA; LIBONATI, 2008).

Despite the impact of lipodystrophy syndrome, little is known about it. Current data suggests that it has a multifactorial etiology, mainly related to the choice of treatment and individual patient factors, and that the risk increases with the duration and type of treatment, patient age, level of immunodeficiency and viral load; and its prevalence, in various studies, has varied between 18% and 83% (SOARES; COSTA, 2013; CECCATO et al., 2011; SEGATTO et al., 2011; DIEHL et al., 2008; DUTRA; LIBONATI, 2008).

HIV infection can have significant effects on physical appearance. Throughout the history of the epidemic, HIV-infected individuals have experienced drastic bodily changes (LEITE; PAPA; VALENTINI, 2011; DUTRA; LIBONATI, 2008).

In PLWHA, the changes in body image caused by lipodystrophy generate dissatisfaction and express the social representation of ART: body image becomes a new stigma because it favors recognition by third parties of the possible positive serological condition for HIV, reducing quality of life and adherence to treatment (PADOIN et al., 2015; SIGNORINI et al., 2012; CECCATO et al., 2011; DUTRA; LIBONATI, 2008).

Lipodystrophy syndrome causes changes in body image, but the most obvious and impacting loss of fat is in the facial region. Facial lipoatrophy causes a reduction in fat in the malar and temporal regions, leading to wrinkling of the face and an appearance of premature ageing (SOARES; COSTA, 2011). These changes in body image and facial physique can trigger TMD.

Psychological alterations frequently associated with HIV and their predictive factors are: mood disorders, depression, stress related to the health-disease process, a history of psychiatric disorders, drug use and suicide in the family. Since social support and the early detection of these factors and the symptoms of psychological disorders, quality of life and adherence to treatment, it can be inferred that social support is essential so that it does not negatively influence adherence to treatment and the quality of life of people with HIV/AIDS (CALVETTI et al., 2014; CAMARGO; CAPITÂO; FILIPE, 2014; TUFANO et al., 2014; BONOLO et al., 2013; SILVEIRA et al., 2012; REIS et al., 2010).

According to Dutra and Libonati (2008), there is currently no standard treatment for lipodystrophy syndrome. However, Segatto et al. (2011) point to nutritional intervention and physical exercise as possibilities for effective interventions to improve physical appearance, prognosis and prevention of cardiovascular diseases.

Thus, the question arose: can the risk of developing lipodystrophic syndrome and depression associated with the diagnosis of HIV/AIDS and the length of time on ART trigger TMD in PLWHA? To this end, the study aimed to identify the risk factors for Temporomandibular Dysfunction, lipodystrophy syndrome and the presence of depression in people living with HIV/AIDS, by: characterizing the study participants in terms of socioeconomic, demographic, habits and lifestyle variables; investigating the prevalence of TMD and depression in the population studied; as well as verifying the association between the risk of lipodystrophy and the presence of TMD and depression in PLWHA.

Considering the size of the population of people living with HIV/AIDS and the complications related to the treatment of the disease, as well as the epidemiology of temporomandibular dysfunction, this study is justified by the epidemic and scientific relevance of these diseases for public health, their social and economic implications and the possible benefits related to knowledge about this problem.

By knowing the risk factors for lipodystrophy syndrome, depression and TMD and their association, it can be determined whether or not the PLWHA population is more vulnerable to developing these disorders.

2. THEORETICAL FRAMEWORK

2.1 TEMPOROMANDIBULAR DYSFUNCTION: conceptual aspects and associated factors

The term temporomandibular disorder (TMD) has been used to define conditions involving craniofacial alterations, the temporomandibular joint (TMJ), the function of the masticatory system or other musculoskeletal structures associated with the head and neck, with a multifactorial or biopsychosocial etiology (DALL' ANTONIA et al., 2013; PASINATO et al., 2011).

The TMJ is considered to be the only mobile joint in the skull and one of the most complete in the human being, as it allows various movements, such as: opening, closing, protrusion, retrusion and laterality of the mandible and, in order for it to function properly, the joint itself, dental occlusion and neuromuscular balance must be harmoniously related (SHARMA et al., 2011; MACHADO et al., 2010).

When these structures are not harmoniously connected, TMD arises, which is responsible for pain and dysfunction in the TMJ and the muscles that control its movement (SHARMA et al., 2011).

TMD can be of articular origin, i.e. those in which the signs and symptoms are related to the TMJ, or of muscular origin, in which the signs and symptoms are related to the stomatognathic musculature (DONNARUMMA et al., 2010).

The causes of TMD are complex and multifactorial. There are numerous factors that can contribute to and increase the risk of TMD or perpetuate it by increasing the progression of the disease or interfering with healing (SHARMA et al., 2011). However, it cannot be said to what extent these factors are considered predisposing or merely coincidental (SANTOS et al., 2006).

Studies point to the following as etiological factors in TMD: poor occlusion, orthodontic treatment, parafunctional habits (bruxism, onychophagia, resting hand on jaw, digital or pacifier sucking), failure to replace missing teeth, trauma, nutritional problems, degenerative or systemic diseases (rheumatoid arthritis, psoriatic arthritis and systemic lupus erythematosus), ligament laxity, exogenous estrogen, stress, tension, anxiety (CALIXTRE et al., 2014; CAMACHO et al., 2014; PIZOLATO; FERNANDES; GAVIÂO, 2013; PASINATO et al., 2011; SHARMA et al., 2011; DONNARUMMA et al., 2010; JANUZZI et al., 2010; MACHADO et al., 2010; MORENO et al., 2009; SANTOS et al., 2006; PEREIRA; DUARTE; VILELA, 2000). In addition to neurophysiological phenomena, psychological, cognitive, behavioral and social aspects are also involved (DALL' ANTONIA et al., 2013).

The main signs and symptoms of TMD are orofacial pain, joint noises (caused by displacements or structural alterations of the joint surface and hypermobility of the condyle-disc complex and degenerative processes), limitation in the range of mandibular movements (opening of the mouth and lateral and protrusive movements or a combination of them), headache, otalgia, ear fullness, hearing loss, perception of tinnitus, vertigo, painful palpation of temporomandibular structures, sleep disorders, asymptomatic radiographic changes (CAMACHO et al., 2014; DALL' ANTONIA et al., 2013; LEITE et al., 2013; ORTEGA; GUIMARÂES, 2013; PIZOLATO; FERNANDES; GAVIÂO, 2013; SENA et al., 2013; ZAVANELLI et al., 2013; PASINATO et al., 2011; MACHADO et al., 2010; DONNARUMMA et al., 2010; MORENO et al., 2009; SANTOS et al., 2006). These include pain, bruxism, depression and stress.

The most common symptom associated with TMD is pain, usually localized in the muscles of mastication, the pre-auricular area and/or TMJ, which can range from incapacitating, intense pain to restriction of movement and distortion of posture. The TMJ and associated structures are considered the most common cause of orofacial pain, as the pain is often aggravated by chewing or other functional activities. Despite the many studies on TMD pain, there are few explanations of its etiology, mechanisms and treatments, but it is known that because it has multifactorial characteristics, its treatment should be multiprofessional (CORREIA et al., 2014; DALL' ANTONIA et al., 2013; LEITE et al., 2013; ZAVANELLI et al., 2013).

Bruxism is a parafunctional oral habit characterized by clenching or grinding teeth and is considered an etiological factor in the onset and perpetuation of TMD. While depression is the emotional state most commonly associated with chronic pain, anxiety can also be associated with TMD because individuals with TMD are more anxious and/or depressed and TMD symptoms begin during periods of psychological stress (anxiety) and are exacerbated during stressful situations, which shows a direct relationship between stress and TMD (CALIXTRE et al., 2014; ORTEGA; GUIMARÂES, 2013; PIZOLATO; FERNANDES; GAVIÂO, 2013; PASINATO et al., 2011; DONNARUMMA et al., 2010; SANTOS et al., 2006).

Ophthalmic symptoms may also be present (photophobia, darkening of vision, tearing, eyelid swelling, conjunctival hyperemia, burning and orbital pain, for example) as the eyes are among the most common sites of pain (20%), as well as the face, throat and neck (PEREIRA; DUARTE; VILELA, 2000).

TMD manifests itself as a group of signs and symptoms that affect a particular population profile. Some variables such as gender and age influence the clinical expression of this condition (MAZZETTO et al., 2014). It is a condition that most often affects adults, although signs and symptoms of TMD have been observed in children (SENA et al., 2013). With regard to the elderly, in a study by Camacho (2014) the elderly showed a high prevalence of TMD, especially in females. However, we must take into account that the variability in the prevalence of TMD may be due to the different types and qualities of analysis methods (SENA et al., 2013).

Several studies have shown a higher frequency of signs and symptoms in women and that they are more severe in this group (MAYORAL; ESPINOSA; MONTIEL, 2013; SENA et al., 2013; SHARMA et al., 2011; DONNARUMMA et al., 2010; MORENO et al., 2009; OLIVEIRA et al., 2006). This is related to neuropsychological factors (women seem to have a lower pain threshold, a higher frequency of psychosomatic illnesses and are more vulnerable to stress) and physiological factors such as hormonal changes (SENA et al., 2013).

In their studies, Mayoral, Espinosa and Montiel (2013) and Sena et al. (2013)

concluded that hormonal variations could be a determining factor because hormones obviously play a role in the etiology, pointing out that there is a higher frequency of TMD at puberty and a reduction in prevalence rates post-menopause. Pereira, Duarte and Vilela (2000) state that the higher incidence of joint noise in women is explained by the fact that the increase in the estrogen hormone can cause generalized flaccidity in the TMJ. Another fact is that among those seeking treatment for TMD, by far the vast majority are women, outnumbering men by at least 4-1 (SHARMA et al., 2011).

With regard to age, Donnarumma et al. (2010) and Bonjardim et al. (2005) showed that the age group with the highest prevalence of TMD is between 20 and 40 years old, and is lower among children, adolescents and the elderly. Mazzetto et al. (2014), in their study, found no correlation between age and the severity of TMD, but observed a trend towards greater severity of symptoms in young adults aged 25-50.

The tissues of the TMJ contain numerous cells with estrogen receptors. These structures can be considered a target for sex steroids, particularly estrogen, which can influence the content and characteristics of collagen fibers. Another possible factor is the hormone relaxin, which is a female hormone produced by the corpus luteum. It appears in the blood during the days before the menstrual cycle, sporadically during the full gestation period and also modulates muscle activity in female reproductive organs (MAYORAL; ESPINOSA; MONTIEL, 2013). Thus, in their study, Mayoral, Espinosa and Montiel (2013) observed that the prevalence of TMD in pregnant women was three times less than in non-pregnant women and concluded that pregnancy is a protective factor against the signs and symptoms of TMD.

Among the tools used to assess TMD are questionnaires, clinical assessment and radiographic, tomographic or magnetic resonance imaging tests, which are used according to the applicability and objectives of the professional (SENA et al., 2013).

But currently, the RDC/TMD (Research diagnostic criteria for temporomandibular disorders) offers the best classification for grouping TMD: the RDC/TMD (Research diagnostic criteria for temporomandibular disorders) allows assessment by means of depression scores and unspecific physical symptoms including or not pain, which represent physical manifestations of anxiety; and muscle disorders, articular disc derangements and painful and degenerative TMJ conditions are classified as distinct diagnostic groups defined by specific criteria, although not mutually exclusive (PASINATO et al., 2011; TESCH; URSI; DENARDIN, 2004).

The RDC/TMD requires a standardized examination, and allows the diagnosis of TMD with three sub-diagnoses: Group I - describes the muscular forms of TMD; Group II - refers to disc displacement; Group III - includes TMD with arthralgia, osteoarthritis and arthrosis. However, despite being the gold standard for diagnosing TMD, we have to be careful when interpreting the results because one of the possible limitations of this diagnostic system is the apparent interrelationship observed between the different diagnostic categories (GONÇALVES et al., 2013; TESCH; URSI; DENARDIN, 2004).

According to Tesch, Ursi and Denardin (2004), there is still a large gap between diagnosis and therapy based on scientific evidence and clinical practice, due in part to the difficulties in recognizing, among the large volume of published literature, which studies are valid and can be applied to the patient's needs.

However, from the available literature, it can be seen that the etiology of TMD can be proven to stem from behavioral and environmental patterns, regardless of the individual's genetics, and are amenable to intervention (ORTEGA; GUIMARÃES, 2013). Thus, according to Januzzi et al. (2010), the most commonly used treatments for TMD control described in the literature are: occlusal plates, occlusal adjustment by selective wear, orthodontic treatment, oral rehabilitation, pharmacotherapy, cognitive behavioral therapy, biofeedback, physiotherapy, surgery and others. Among these treatments, occlusal appliances and occlusal adjustment are the most widespread and used by clinicians.

Dall'Antonia et al. (2013) cite botulinum toxin type A as a possible treatment for myofascial pain, as it has been the subject of studies into pain control and is related to the pain-relieving mechanism, but conclude that this method is no more efficient than conventional treatments, as there are few studies with good evidence and many controversies regarding its effectiveness.

Although orthodontic treatments are the most widely used in the treatment of TMD, scholars claim that there is no association between orthodontic treatment, occlusion and TMD, and that occlusal adjustment and orthodontic treatment should not be indicated to treat or prevent TMD, because they do not present adequate efficacy and safety, in addition to the lack of evidence of their benefits (ORTEGA; GUIMARÃES, 2013; JANUZZI et al., 2010; BÓSIO, 2004). As for the occlusal appliance for nighttime use, good quality evidence points to it as a safe intervention for controlling myofascial pain, both in the short (75 days) and long (365 days) term (JANUZZI et al., 2010).

Leite et al. (2013), in their study, state that from the studies found in the literature review, orthodontic treatment, regardless of the technique used, does not increase the signs and symptoms of TMD and is therefore not a risk factor for its development. Orthodontic treatment does not appear to be a valuable resource for treating or preventing the onset of TMD signs and symptoms. There is a need to improve the methodology used in studies that seek to demonstrate the association between TMD and orthodontic treatment so that they can be less contradictory.

Two important parts of effective treatment are early diagnosis and multi-professional treatment (dentist, psychologist and physiotherapist are among the most cited) (ZAVANELLI et al., 2013; BONJARDIM et al., 2005). Still according to Zavanelli et al. (2013), the individual must be analyzed as a whole, investigating their biopsychosocial aspects, surveying all the factors that may be involved in the onset of the disease, so that treatment can achieve the expected result.

Taking into account the most varied aspects of TMD (etiological factors, symptoms, diagnosis and treatment) it can be inferred that this is a disease with a picture of signs and symptoms whose relationship is not yet well defined; that the importance of certain etiological factors is not yet well measured despite the fact that stress and female gender are widely cited in various studies; that the diagnostic criteria for TMD have dubious points; and, that the treatment used to date is still not what would be ideal for the disease due to the lack of significant evidence on the subject and an attitude of trial and error on the part of professionals because what works for one patient may not work for another, without taking into account the placebo factor of these treatments.

2.2 DEPRESSION IN PEOPLE LIVING WITH HIV/AIDS

Chronic diseases can cause or aggravate mental disorders, either as an individual response to the disease, by affecting immunity, or as a side effect of treatment. Most HIV-infected patients are diagnosed with one or more mental disorders, a rate two to three times higher than that of the general population. The most frequent are mood disorders, anxiety disorders, psychotic disorders or alcohol and drug abuse (TUFANO et al., 2015; GUIMARÀES et al., 2014).

The treatment of people living with HIV/AIDS can provoke psychological reactions such as anxiety and depression. Anxiety is related to uncertainties about the evolution of the disease, treatment and death. Depression is associated with negative beliefs about the disease and feelings of hopelessness (CALVETTI et al., 2014).

Depression is commonly experienced by people with chronic diseases, causing disability, affecting the progression of the disease and interfering with recovery, and is a potential risk for increased morbidity and mortality in these people. Among the various psychiatric disorders identified in people living with HIV/AIDS, depression is the most prevalent (REIS et al., 2011).

Older people living with HIV may be more prone to faster clinical and immunological deterioration during ART and may have chronic comorbidities. Studies have found that HIV patients may be at greater risk of developing depression and that a diagnosis of depression is associated with low adherence to ART (CARMO FILHO et al., 2013).

Mental disorders are known to be triggers of great psychic suffering and also predisposing factors for suicide attempts. Therefore, the comorbidity of mental disorders with infectious diseases, such as HIV/AIDS, has to be properly investigated and managed to increase therapeutic effectiveness and prevent complications (GUIMARÂES et al., 2014).

Studies on quality of life among people living with HIV/AIDS point out that it is affected by numerous individual, cultural, social and emotional factors, related to the impact of diagnosis and treatment and living with a chronic illness, and that depression affects all dimensions of quality of life and is closely related to it, especially in individuals with chronic illnesses (REIS et al., 2011).

Diagnosing and treating these symptoms is fundamental to improving patients' quality of life. However, 50% to 60% of cases go undiagnosed (SILVEIRA et al., 2012).

It is therefore important for health professionals to understand the role of psychosocial aspects such as stress, anxiety, depression and social support in adhering to treatment and improving quality of life. As the survival rate of PLWHA increases and the fear of imminent death decreases, these people begin to feel the need to return to their routine and maintain their relationships with family, community and work, as well as forming new relationships (CALVETTI et al., 2014).

2.3 LIPODYSTROPHIC SYNDROME AND ANTIRETROVIRAL THERAPY IN people living with HIV/AIDS

Initially, the advent of HIV infection and the development of AIDS was linked to homosexuals, injecting drug users and hemophiliacs, but the epidemiology and initial trends of infection/transmission have changed over time. The idea of the existence of specific risk groups gave way to the idea of risk behaviors and, later, vulnerability (pADoiN et al., 2015; CAMARGo; CApiTAo; FiLipE, 2014).

However, what seemed to be a male-only pattern was de-characterized throughout the 1990s, due to the rapid emergence of infection among women. Over the last decade, the profile of infected Brazilians has shifted from middle- to upper-class urban men to poor women, a fact that has led to changes in the epidemiological profile of AIDS and has been called the feminization of the epidemic (pADoiN et al., 2015; EiRA et al., 2012; FELiX; CEoLiM, 2012).

However, according to Moraes, Oliveira and Costa (2014), since 2008 the number of cases of AIDs in young men has been increasing at a faster rate than in women, rising from 0.9 cases in men for every woman (2000-2005) to 1.9 cases in men for every case in women (2012). Furthermore, in Brazil there has been a 67.8% increase in the detection of cases in young men and a 12.2% decrease in young women.

HIV infection is a major public health problem in Brazil and worldwide. At the beginning of the epidemic, the life expectancy of people living with HIV was minimal. Since 1996, with the advent of Highly Active Antiretroviral Therapy (HAART), the course of the disease has undergone profound changes and there has been an increase in survival and improvement in quality of life (reduction in morbidity and mortality), as well as partial restoration of the immune system (increase in CD4 lymphocytes and reduction in HIV viral load, which can be undetectable) (CAMARGO; CApITAo; FILIpE, 2014; sILVA et al., 2014; TUFANo et al., 2014; ARMENTANo et al., 2013; BONOLO et al., 2013; FUKUMOTO et al., 2013; DOMINGOS et al., 2012; EIRA et al., 2012; FELIX; CEOLIM, 2012; GODOI et al..., 2012; KROLL et al., 2012; ROMANCINI et al., 2012; ROSSI et al., 2012; OLIVEIRA; OLIVEIRA; SOUZA, 2011; SEGATTO et al., 2011; VIANA et al., 2011; REIS et al., 2010; DUTRA; LIBONATI, 2008).

To achieve this desired clinical effect, adherence to the HAART regimen is necessary (CAMARGO; CAPITAO; FILIPE, 2014; MORAES; OLIVEIRA; COSTA, 2014; TUFANO et al., 2014; FELIX; CEOLIM, 2012; REIS et al., 2010). Currently, initial therapy should include at least three drugs: two nucleotide reverse transcriptase inhibitors associated with a non-nucleotide reverse transcriptase inhibitor or a protease inhibitor, preferably with the administration of ritonavir to increase pharmacokinetics (FUKUMOTO et al., 2013). Non-adherence to treatment results in persistent viral replication, viral resistance and failure of the therapeutic project (CAMARGO; CAPITAO; FILIPE, 2014; MORAES; OLIVEIRA; COSTA, 2014;

FELIX; CEOLIM, 2012; LEITE; PAPA; VALENTINI, 2011).

Today, about 10 years into the use of HAART, adverse effects are beginning to appear in the body. These include changes in lipid metabolism leading to hypertriglyceridemia, hypercholesterolemia and other metabolic changes such as insulin resistance, hyperglycemia and redistribution of body fat (lipodystrophy), leading to increased arterial stiffness and the incidence of myocardial infarction. All of these changes are known as Human Immunodeficiency Virus Lipodystrophy Syndrome (HIV-LS) or HIV Lipodystrophy Syndrome (HIVLS) (ARMENTANO et al., 2013; SOARES; COSTA, 2013; DOMINGOS et al., 2012; EIRA et al., 2012; GODOI et al., 2012; ROMANCINI et al., 2012; ANJOS et al., 2011; CECCATO et al., 2011; SEGATTO et al., 2011; DUTRA; LIBONATI, 2008).

According to Romancini et al. (2012), the lipid changes found include factors that contribute to the origin of atheromatous plaques, and the use of ART for more than 10 years implies a 100% probability of developing lipodystrophy (redistribution of peripheral fat to the central region, mainly abdominal).

Oliveira, Oliveira and Souza (2011) draw attention to the most immediate adverse effects of ART and their importance for adherence to treatment. These are: gastric intolerance, nausea, vomiting, abdominal pain, asthenia, headache or insomnia.

Among the multiple causes of non-adherence to ART, we can observe: social factors (age, race, gender, income, marital status and schooling), behavioral factors (use of alcohol and drugs), psychological factors (anxiety, stress, depression), clinical factors (adverse effects of treatment and changes in body image) and health service factors (health team-patient relationship and access to services) (GALVAO et al.., 2015; PADOIN et al., 2015; CALVETTI et al., 2014; CAMARGO et al., 2014; MORAES; OLIVEIRA; COSTA, 2014; TUFANO et al., 2014; BONOLO et al., 2013; KROLL et al., 2012; SILVEIRA et al., 2012; LEITE; PAPA; VALENTINI, 2011; REIS et al., 2010).

Galvao et al. (2015) concluded in their study that people at the beginning of HIV treatment have inadequate levels of adherence to antiretroviral drugs and it is possible that they have suffered losses in quality of life and adherence because they are adapting to a new life condition.

With regard to the adverse effects of ART, the ones most cited by the authors are physical (metabolic and nutritional changes, increased cardiovascular risk and lipodystrophy) and psychological (anxiety, depression and stress).

Metabolic alterations are risk factors associated with the development of cardiovascular diseases and, despite the impact of the lipodystrophy syndrome, little is known about its pathogenesis, prevention, diagnosis and treatment or even a precise definition of lipodystrophy. However, current data suggests a multifactorial etiology, mainly related to the choice of treatment and the patient's individual characteristics, and that the risk increases with the duration and type of treatment, the patient's age, level of immunodeficiency and viral load (SOARES; COSTA, 2013; CECCATO et al., 2011; SEGATTO et al., 2011; DIEHL et al., 2008; DUTRA; LIBONATI, 2008).

HIV infection can have significant effects on physical appearance. Throughout the history of the epidemic, HIV-infected individuals have experienced drastic bodily changes, ranging from severe malnutrition to lipodystrophy and reaching a significant increase in the prevalence of overweight (LEITE; PAPA; VALENTINI, 2011; DUTRA; LIBONATI, 2008).

In their study, Kroll et al. (2012) observed that among the patients studied, overweight was the most common nutritional disorder, especially among women, as occurs in the Brazilian population in general, but they found no statistically significant association between the findings and the use or not of therapy.

The changes in body image caused by lipodystrophy generate dissatisfaction and express the social representation of ART: body image becomes a new stigma because it favors recognition by third parties of the possible HIV-positive serological condition; decreasing quality of life and adherence to treatment (PADOIN et al., 2015; CECCATO et al., 2011; DUTRA; LIBONATI, 2008). Leite, Papa and Valentini (2011) observed in their study a high prevalence of irregular adherence among those dissatisfied with their body image and suggest multidisciplinary approaches to reduce dissatisfaction and increase self-esteem, as well as other less conventional actions aimed at aesthetics, health and beauty, with a view to strengthening adherence, especially among women.

All those involved in caring for these patients, especially nurses, must recognize the signs of the lipodystrophy syndrome, as well as the indicated treatments to be incorporated into their therapeutic regimes. Among the anatomical changes caused by fat redistribution, for example, we can observe: lipoatrophy, lipohypertrophy and mixed forms. In lipohypertrophy, there is central or localized fat accumulation in the abdomen, neck, back, breasts and other areas. In lipoatrophy, there is a peripheral loss of subcutaneous tissue in the upper and lower limbs, and the skin becomes thinner, allowing muscle groups and superficial blood vessels to be seen. The mixed form is a combination of lipoatrophy and lipohypertrophy (SOARES; COSTA, 2011).

Armentano et al. (2013) grouped the main changes related to lipodystrophy into three categories: psychosocial changes (difficulties in social and sexual relationships, loss of self-esteem and social isolation), bodily changes (central lipohypertrophy, peripheral lipoatrophy and mixed lipodystrophy) and metabolic abnormalities (hypertriglyceridemia, hypercholesterolemia, mixed dyslipidemia, insulin resistance and/or type 2 diabetes mellitus).

Also according to Soares and Costa (2011; 2013) and Signorini et al. (2012), changes in body image can be extremely disturbing in terms of psychosocial well-being, especially when it comes to facial lipodystrophy which, because it is more apparent, is responsible for the greater stigmatization of HIV/AIDS sufferers and leads to psychological problems, social and family relationships, isolation and abandonment of treatment, directly impacting on their quality of life.

Facial lipoatrophy consists of the progressive loss of facial adipose tissue, mainly in the malar and temporal regions. As a consequence, furrows and depressions develop in the skin and expression lines become more prominent, resulting in a skeletal and aged appearance. (SOARES; COSTA, 2013)

According to Dutra and Libonati (2008), there is currently no standard treatment for lipodystrophy syndrome and the decision on which treatment to adopt will depend on a number of variables: symptoms, clinical picture, type of ART, length of use and the presence of one or more cardiovascular risk factors. However, together with Segatto et al. (2011), they point to nutritional intervention and physical exercise as possibilities for effective interventions to improve physical appearance, prognosis and prevention of cardiovascular diseases.

Regarding psychological changes, Camargo, Capitao and Filipe (2014) state that some classic psychiatric syndromes, such as mood disorders, and particularly depression, are often associated with HIV and that the associated predictive factors are a history of psychiatric disorders (particularly depression), drug use and suicide in the family. The psychological changes are due to the life circumstances associated with the HIV diagnosis, such as unemployment, abandonment or family breakdown and feelings of guilt or fear of pain and death. They also highlight other diagnoses or symptoms: adaptation or adjustment disorders, insomnia, dependence on or abuse of alcohol and other drugs and psychotic disorders.

The study by Calvetti et al. (2014) revealed a correlation between social support, quality of life and adherence to treatment, where it can be inferred that social support is essential for moderating stress related to the health-disease process, involving issues such as fear of death, abandonment by family and friends, unemployment and responsibilities related to being HIV positive.

Nursing therefore plays an important role in the early detection of possible indicators of symptoms of psychological disorders with the aim of palliating or treating them so that they do not negatively influence adherence to treatment and the quality of life of people with HIV/AIDS, as well as strategies for clinical and social interventions and facilitating access to health services (TUFANO et al., 2014; BONOLO et al., 2013; SILVEIRA et al., 2012; REIS et al., 2010).

Therefore, we can see common aspects between the consequences of the lipodystrophy syndrome and the etiological factors of TMD, where the symptoms of one can be triggering factors for the other.

3. METHODOLOGY

3.1 TYPE OF STUDY

This was a descriptive, exploratory, cross-sectional study with a quantitative approach, developed by applying questionnaires to people living with HIV/AIDS in clinical and outpatient care.

A descriptive study aims to describe reality without intervening in it and is fundamental when little is known about a particular subject (ARAGÂO, 2011). Exploratory studies aim to provide greater familiarity with the problem, its classification and definition in order to make it more explicit (GIL, 2007).

The cross-sectional study describes a phenomenon at an undefined time, only represented by the presence of a disease or disorder, examining the sample members for the presence or absence of exposure or the effects of the disease (HOCHMAN et al., 2005).

A quantitative approach means that the data and results obtained from the research are quantified in order to describe the causes of a phenomenon and the relationships between the variables using mathematics, and the samples used are generally large and can be considered representative of the population (FONSECA, 2002).

3.2 STUDY SETTING

The study was carried out in a Specialized Assistance Service (SAE) located in the city of Caxias - MA, as it is a reference center for people living with HIV/AIDS.

The Specialized Assistance Service (SAE) is an outpatient clinic integrated into the SUS, designed to monitor STD/HIV/AIDS patients and aims to provide specialized assistance to these individuals, as well as carrying out specific tests and distributing the necessary medication (SILVA; TAKAHASHI, 2008; OLIVEIRA, 2014).

3.3 POPULATION AND SAMPLE

The study's reference population consisted of the 421 HIV-positive people registered with the SAE. Sampling was of the non-probabilistic accidental type, since it consisted of the subjects who attended the SAE during the data collection period.

In order to be included in the study, the individuals had to meet the following criteria: be aged 18 or over; have a positive HIV test result, whether or not they had developed the Syndrome; be using antiretroviral therapy; be at the SAE at the time of data collection; be physically, mentally and psychologically able to take part in the interview; and agree to take part in the study.

Thus, the following were excluded from the study: individuals under the age of 18; those who did not attend the SAE during the data collection period; those not using ART; pregnant women; and those who did not agree to take part in the study.

3.4 INSTRUMENTS AND DATA COLLECTION

Data collection took place from September to November 2015, through the application of questionnaires to PLWHA who attended the data collection site during the collection period. They are:

A) Anthropometric assessment questionnaire, aspects of HIV infection, self-reported lipodystrophy, body image and lifestyle habits (Annex A)

This is an instrument adapted from others that were previously used in the study by Soares (2011) and Justina (2013) and was used in the research as shown in the annex

A. It consists of semi-open and closed questions on the following variables: personal and socio-economic data, anthropometric assessment, aspects of HIV infection and ART, individuals' perception of changes in the distribution of adipose tissue and body image, and lifestyle habits.

B) Fonseca instrument for TMD assessment (Appendix B)

The clinical index by Fonseca et al. (1994) is made up of 10 closed questions with three alternatives and is used to classify individuals by level of TMD severity, where the participant has to mark only one answer. After completing the questionnaire, the alternatives were added up (each alternative has a score) to classify them as: no temporomandibular dysfunction (0 to 15 points); mild dysfunction (20 to 40 points); moderate dysfunction (45 to 65 points) and severe dysfunction (70 to 100 points), according to Fonseca's index.

This instrument was developed along the lines of Helkimo's (1974) anamnestic index, and is one of the few instruments available in Portuguese to characterize the severity of TMD symptoms (CHAVES; OLIVEIRA; GROSSI, 2008).

C)   Beck Depression Inventory (BDI)

The Beck Depression Inventory (BDI) was developed by Beck and colleagues in 1961 to assess the intensity of depression and, according to its authors, it proved to be a highly reliable instrument. It was translated into Portuguese in 1982 and validated by Gorenstein & Andrade (1996) (MALUF, 2002).

The BDI is made up of 21 categories containing alternatives that express the levels of severity of depressive symptoms. The score for each category ranges from 0 to 3, where 0 is the absence of symptoms and 3 is the presence of the most intense symptoms. With regard to the total score (the sum of the scores for each category), scores of up to 9 points signify the absence of depression or minimal depressive symptoms; from 10 to

18 points, mild to moderate depression; 19 to 29 points, moderate to severe depression; and 30 to 63, severe depression (MALUF, 2002).

3.5 DATA ANALYSIS

The data was analyzed by constructing yes and relative frequencies. Fisher's exact test was used to test for associations between the study variables, and the free software R version 3.0.2 was used to carry out the tests. The tables and graphs were drawn up using Excel. The level of statistical significance adopted for the tests was $p<0.05$.

3.6 ETHICAL ASPECTS

The project for this study was sent to the Brazil Platform for submission to a Research Ethics Committee (CEP) for approval. The researcher in charge has committed himself to the standards set out in Resolution No.[0] 466 of December 12, 2012, published on June 13, 2013, guaranteeing research participants respect, anonymity and confidentiality of the data collected, as well as the freedom to refuse to participate in the research or to stop participating at any time without any harm to the participant, among others contained in the Informed Consent Form (ICF) (Appendix A).

The risks of this study were minimal, including the possibility of embarrassment and/or discomfort in relation to some of the questions in the questionnaire, such as the alternatives in the Beck Depression Scale, and the identification of being HIV-positive. The study participants did not benefit directly, but the results could have a positive influence on the health of all PLHIV, as well as on the quality of care provided.

4. RESULTS

In order to achieve the aim of this study, the results were divided into seven parts: 1. characterization of the participants in terms of socio-economic variables, habits and lifestyle; 2. characterization of self-reported lypodystrophy; 3. prevalence of TMD; 4. prevalence of depression; 5. association between lypodystrophy and TMD; 6. association between lypodystrophy and the presence of TMD. Prevalence of TMD; 4. Prevalence of depression; 5. Association between self-reported lypodystrophy and the presence of TMD; 6. Association between self-reported lypodystrophy and the presence of depression; 7. Association between the presence of TMD and depression.

4.1 CHARACTERIZATION OF PARTICIPANTS IN TERMS OF SOCIOECONOMIC, DEMOGRAPHIC, HABITS AND LIFESTYLE VARIABLES

Table 1 shows the socio-economic and demographic characteristics of the sample studied. With regard to gender, the individuals were equally distributed between female (50%) and male (50%). The predominant color was brown (65.63%), followed by black (18.75%). The majority of the individuals studied were from Caxias (53.13%), while the rest were from other municipalities. The most frequent level of schooling was incomplete primary education (43.75%), 21.88% had completed primary education and the remaining percentage was distributed between illiterate (12.5%), completed secondary education (12.5%) and incomplete secondary education (9.38%). More than half of the sample is single (56.25%), 31.25% married, 9.38% widowed and 3.13% divorced. The sample is generally made up of low-income individuals, with 87.5% earning 1 minimum wage or less.

Table 2 shows the habits and lifestyle of the sample surveyed. It shows that 65.63% had smoked at some time and, at the time of the survey, 47.62% said they were still smoking. The majority of smokers had been using cigarettes for more than 10 years (64.71%) and 35.29% had been smoking for 10 years or less. A large proportion had already consumed alcohol (87.5%) and 53.57% currently consume alcohol. The majority of drinkers had been drinking for between 10 and 20 years (40%), 32% for more than 20 years and 28% for less than 10 years. With regard to the number of daily meals, 40.63% eat 3 or 4 meals a day and 59.38% eat 5 or 6 meals a day. Only 25% of the sample practiced some kind of physical exercise.

Table 1 - Socioeconomic and demographic characterization of the sample. Caxias- MA, 2015 (n=32).

Variable	N	%
Sex		
Female	16	50,00
Male	16	50,00
Color		
White	3	9,38
Brown	21	65,63
Yellow	2	6,25
Black	6	18,75
Naturalness		
Caxias	17	53,13
Gold municipality	15	46,88
Education		
Illiterate	4	12,50
Elementary school incomplete	14	43,75
Complete primary education	7	21,88
High school incomplete	3	9,38
Complete high school	4	12,50
Marital status		
Single	18	56,25
Married	10	31,25
Divorced	1	3,13
Viùvo	3	9,38
Occupation		
Unemployed	8	25,00
Employee	24	75,00
Family income		
Up to 1 minimum wage	28	87,50
2 or 3 minimum wages	4	12,50

Table 2 - Distribution of habits and lifestyle of the individuals in the sample. Caxias - MA, 2015.

Variable	N	%
Ever smoked (n=32)		
Yes	21	65,63
No	11	34,38
Current smoker (n=21)		
Yes	10	47,62
No	11	52,38

Keep going...

Table 2 - Distribution of the Imbits and lifestyle of the individuals in the sample. Caxias - MA, 2015.

Variable	N	%
Length of time smoking (n=17)		
10 years or less	6	35,29
More than 10 years	11	64,71
Have you ever drunk alcohol (n=32)		
Yes	28	87,50
No	4	12,50
Currently consumes alcohol (n=28)		
Yes	15	53,57
No	13	46,43
Length of time drinking alcohol (n=25)		
10 years or less	7	28,00
Between 10 and 20 years	10	40,00
More than 20 years	8	32,00
Number of meals per day (n=32)		
3 or 4 meals	13	40,63
5 or 6 meals	19	59,38
Physical exercise (n=32)		
Yes	8	25,00
No	24	75,00

Conclusion

4.2 CHARACTERIZATION OF SELF-REPORTED LIPODYSTROPHY

Table 3 refers to the characterization of self-reported lipodystrophy, anthropometric assessment and general aspects of HIV infection. It can be seen that 56.25% were of normal weight, 31.25% were overweight and 12.50% were underweight. More than 80% of the patients noticed some kind of change in their body, in the face (65.63%), arms (56.25%), neck (6.25%), breasts/chest (53.13%), waist (75%), buttocks (40.63%), thighs (50%), appearance of veins in the arms and legs (81.25%) and presence of lipomas (12.50%). With regard to self-assessment of appearance, 87.50% gave their appearance a score higher than 5.

Table 3 - Characterization of self-reported lipodystrophy, anthropometric assessment and general aspects of HIV. Caxias - MA, 2015.

Features	N	%
BMI		
Low weight	4	12,50
Normal weight	18	56,25
Overweight	10	31,25
Change in body (n=32)		
Changed	26	81,25
It hasn't changed	6	18,75
Change in face (n=32)		
Yes	21	65,63
No	11	34,38
Type of change (n=21)		
Loss of facial fat	12	57,14
Increased cheek size	9	42,86
Change in arms (n=32)		
Yes	18	56,25
No	14	43,75
Type of change (n=18)		
Fat loss in the arms	11	61,11
Increased arm thickness	7	38,89
Change in neck (n=32)		
Yes	2	6,25
No	30	93,75
Breast/chest changes (n=32)		
Yes	17	53,13
No	15	46,88

Type of alteration (n=17)		
Breast/chest reduction	6	35,29
Breast augmentation	11	64,71
Change in waist thickness (n=32)		
Yes	24	75,00
No	8	25,00
Type of change (n=24)		
Decrease	6	25,00
Increase	18	75,00
Change in buttocks (n=32)		
Yes	13	40,63
No	19	59,38
Type of change (n=13)		
Minor/flabby	8	61,54
More	5	38,46

Keep going...

Table 3 - Characterization of self-reported lipodystrophy, anthropometric assessment and aspects

general HIV. Caxias - MA, 2015.

Features	N	%
Change in thighs (n=32)		
Yes	16	50,00
No	16	50,00
Type of change (n=16)		
Fat loss	10	62,50
Increase in size	6	37,50
Change in the appearance of veins in the arms and legs (n=32)		
Yes	26	81,25
No	6	18,75
Type of change (n=26)		
Less visible veins	10	38,46
More visible veins	16	61,54
Presence of lipomas (n=32)		
Yes	4	12,50
No	28	87,50

Appearance score (n=32)

5 or less	4	12,50
More than 5	28	87,50

Conclusion

4.3 PREVALENCE OF TEMPOROMANDIBULAR DISORDERS

Figure 1 summarizes the TMD scale applied to people living with HIV.

The majority had mild dysfunction (53.13%), 31.25% had no dysfunction, 12.5% had moderate dysfunction and only 3.13% had severe dysfunction.

Figure 1 - Prevalence of Temporomandibular Dysfunction in People Living with HIV/AIDS. Caxias - MA, 2015.

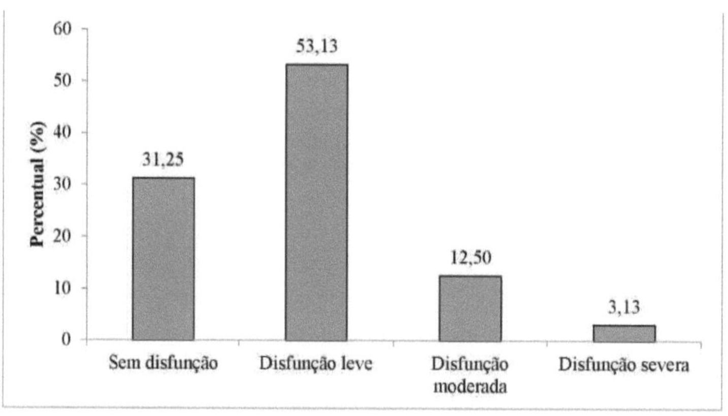

4.4 PREVALENCE OF DEPRESSION

Figure 2 categorically shows the prevalence of depression among the survey subjects. It can be seen that 21.88% do not have depression, 40.63% have mild or moderate depression, 28.13% have moderate to severe depression and 9.38% have severe depression.

Figure 2 - Prevalence of Depression in People Living with HIV/AIDS. Caxias - MA, 2015.

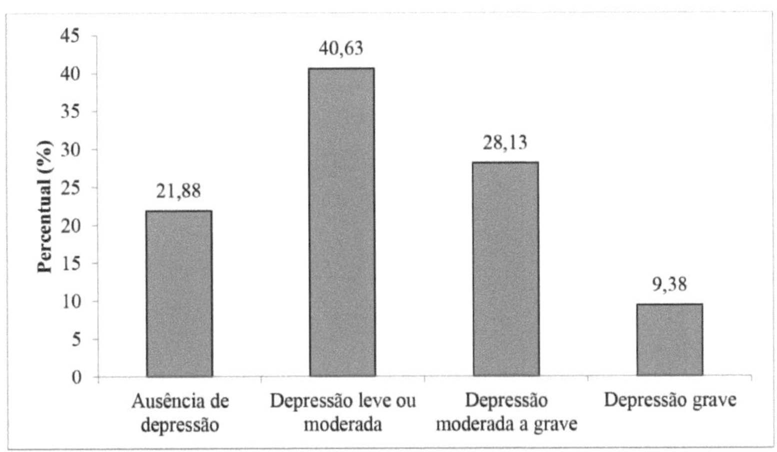

4.5 ASSOCIATION BETWEEN SELF-REPORTED LIPODYSTROPHY AND THE PRESENCE OF TEMPOROMANDIBULAR DISORDER

Table 4 shows the characteristics of self-reported lipodystrophy, anthropometric assessment and general aspects of HIV, according to the presence of TMD. Fisher's test showed that there was no statistical association between the variables self-reported lipodystrophy, anthropometric assessment and general aspects of HIV and TMD (p>0.05).

Table 4 - Association between self-reported hypodystrophy, anthropometric assessment and general aspects of HIV and TMD. Caxias-MA, 2015.

Variable	With dysfunction		No dysfunction		p-value
	n	%	n	%	
BMI (n=32)					
Low weight	3	75,00	1	25,00	
Normal weight	13	72,22	5	27,78	0,767
Overweight	6	60,00	4	40,00	
Change in body (n=32)					
Changed	18	69,23	8	30,77	0,999
It hasn't changed	4	66,67	2	33,33	
Change in face (n=32)					
Yes	16	76,19	5	23,81	0,252
No	6	54,55	5	45,45	

Type of change (n=21)					
Loss of facial fat	10	83,33	2	16,67	0,611
Increased cheek size	6	66,67	3	33,33	
Change in arms (n=32)					
Yes	13	72,22	5	27,78	0,712
No	9	64,29	5	35,71	
Type of change (n=18)					
Fat loss in the arms	8	72,73	3	27,27	0,999
Increased arm thickness	5	71,43	2	28,57	
Change in neck (n=32)					
Yes	2	100,00	0	0,00	
No	20	66,67	10	33,33	
Breast changes (n=32)					
Yes	12	70,59	5	29,41	0,999
No	10	66,67	5	33,33	
Type of alteration (n=17)					
Breast/chest reduction	5	83,33	1	16,67	0,600
Breast augmentation	7	63,64	4	36,36	
Change in waist thickness (n=32)					
Yes	15	62,50	9	37,50	0,380
No	7	87,50	1	12,50	
Type of change (n=24)					
Decrease	3	50,00	3	50,00	0,635
Increase	12	66,67	6	33,33	
Change in buttocks (n=32)					
Yes	10	76,92	3	23,08	0,467
No	12	63,16	7	36,84	
Type of change (n=13)					
Minor/flabby	7	87,50	1	12,50	0,511
More	3	60,00	2	40,00	
Change in thighs (n=32)					
Yes	10	62,50	6	37,50	0,704
No	12	75,00	4	25,00	

Keep going...

Table 4 - Association between self-reported hypodystrophy, anthropometric assessment and general aspects of HIV and TMD. Caxias-MA, 2015.

Variable	With dysfunction		No dysfunction		p-value
	n	%	n	%	
Type of change (n=16)					
Fat loss	7	70,00	3	30,00	0,607
Increase in size		350,00	3	50,00	
Change in the appearance of the	**arms and legs (n=32)**				
Yes	20	76,92	6	23,08	0,060
No	2	33,33	4	66,67	
Type of change (n=26)					
Less visible veins	7	70,00	3	30,00	0,644
More visible veins	13	81,25	3	18,75	
Presence of lipomas (n=32)					
Yes	3	75,00	1	25,00	0,999
No	19	67,86	9	32,14	
Line Labels (n=32)					
5 or less	2	50,00	2	50,00	0,572
More than 5	20	71,43	8	28,57	

Conclusion

4.6 ASSOCIATION BETWEEN SELF-REPORTED LIPODYSTROPHY AND THE PRESENCE OF DEPRESSION

Table 5 shows the characteristics of self-reported lipodystrophy, anthropometric assessment and general aspects of HIV related to depression. The variables self-reported lipodystrophy, anthropometric assessment and general aspects of HIV were not associated with depression (p>0.05).

Table 5 - Association of self-reported lipodystrophy, anthropometric assessment and general aspects of HIV with depression. Caxias - MA, 2015.

Variables	With depression		No depression		p-value
	n	%	n	%	
Weight (n=29)	3	75,00	1	25,00	
Low weight	15	83,33	3	16,67	0,706
Normal weight	7	70,00	3	30,00	
Overweight	3	75,00	1	25,00	
Change in body (n=32)					

	22	84,62	4	15,38	
Changed	22	84,62	4	15,38	0,101
It hasn't changed	3	50,00	3	50,00	
Change in face (n=32)					
Yes	17	80,95	4	19,05	0,6675
No	8	72,73	3	27,27	

Keep going...

Table 5 - Association of self-reported lipodystrophy, anthropometric assessment and general aspects of HIV with depression. Caxias - MA, 2015.

Variables	With depression		No depression		p-value
	n	%	n	%	
Type of change (n=21)					
Loss of facial fat	10	83,33	2	16,67	0,999
Increased cheek size	7	77,78	2	22,22	
Change in arms (n=32)					
Yes	15	83,33	3	16,67	0,669
No	10	71,43	4	28,57	
Type of change (n=18)					
Fat loss in the arms	9	81,82	2	18,18	0,999
Increased arm thickness	6	85,71	1	14,29	
Change in neck (n=32)					
Yes	2	100,00	0	0,00	
No	23	76,67	7	23,33	--
Breast changes (n=32)					
Yes	13	76,47	4	23,53	0,999
No	12	80,00	3	20,00	
Type of alteration (n=17)					
Breast/chest reduction	5	83,33	1	16,67	0,999
Breast augmentation	8	72,73	3	27,27	
Change in waist thickness (n=32)					
Yes	17	70,83	7	29,17	0,999
No	8	100,00	0	0,00	
Type of change (n=24)					
Decrease	4	66,67	2	33,33	0,999
Increase	13	72,22	5	27,78	
Change in buttocks (n=32)					
Yes	11	84,62	2	15,38	0,971

Variables	n	%	n	%	p-value
No	14	73,68	5	26,32	
Type of change (n=13)					
Minor/flabby	7	87,50	1	12,50	0,999
More	4	80,00	1	20,00	
Change in thighs (n=32)					
Yes	13	81,25	3	18,75	0,999
No	12	75,00	4	25,00	
Type of change (n=16)					
Fat loss	8	80,00	2	20,00	0,999
Increase in	size583	.33	1	16,67	
Change in the appearance of veins in the arms and legs (n=32)					
Yes	22	84,62	4	15,38	0,999
No	3	50,00	3	50,00	

Keep going...

Table 5 - Association of self-reported lipodystrophy, anthropometric assessment and general aspects of HIV with depression. Caxias - MA, 2015.

Variables	With depression		No depression		p-value
	n	%	n	%	
Type of change (n=26)					
Less visible veins	8	80,00	2	20,00	0,999
More visible veins	14	87,50	2	12,50	
Presence of lipomas (n=32)					
Yes	3	75,00	1	25,00	0,999
No	22	78,57	6	21,43	
Appearance (n=32)					
5 or less	3	75,00	1	25,00	0,999
More than 5	22	78,57	6	21,43	

Conclusion

4.7 ASSOCIATION BETWEEN THE PRESENCE OF TEMPOROMANDIBULAR DYSFUNCTION AND DEPRESSION

Figure 3 shows the association between TMD and depression in HIV patients. Fisher's association test showed that TMD was associated with depression ($p=0.001$). Among the individuals without depression (60%), the percentage of individuals with

TMD was 4.55% and, in the group with depression (40%), the percentage of individuals with mild to severe TMD was 95.45%, i.e. individuals with depression are more likely to develop TMD.

Figure 3 - Association between dysfunction and depression in HIV patients. Caxias - MA, 2015.

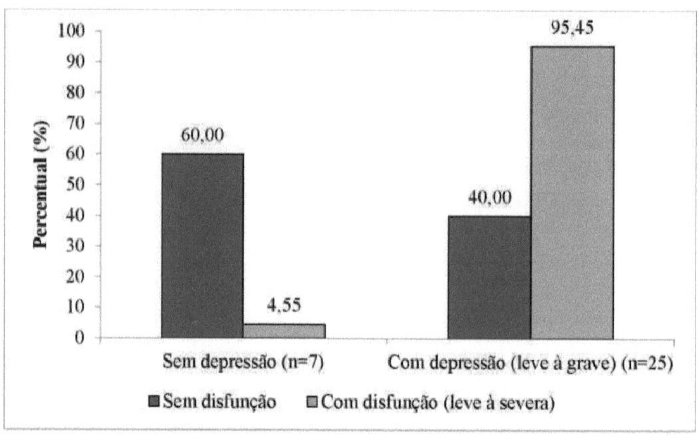

5. Discussion

In the last decade, Brazil has seen an increase in the detection rate of AIDS cases among young men and a reduction among young women, which could result in an increase in the number of men living with HIV/AIDS in the coming years. In addition, it is worth emphasizing that the model of masculinity imposed by society contributes to men not taking on the necessary behavioral changes to prevent transmission of the virus (MORAES; OLIVEIRA; COSTA, 2014).

In this study, the individuals were equally distributed between female (50%) and male (50%). However, in previous studies, men made up the majority of the samples, with a frequency varying between 54.6% and 80% (GALVÂO et al., 2015; KROLL et al., 2012; ROSSI et al., 2012; SIGNORINI et al., 2012; ANJOS et al., 2011; SEGATTO et al., 2011; DIEHL et al., 2008).

Regarding race, the predominant color was brown (65.63%), as in the study by Moraes, Oliveira and Costa (2014) carried out in the state of Pernambuco, where brown individuals represented 52.2% of the sample and, diverging from the study by Kroll et al. (2012) carried out in Porto Alegre, in which the majority of the sample (78.5%) was white.

The divergence between the most predominant race/ethnicity among individuals can be explained by the historical circumstances and colonization of each region of Brazil, which despite being composed of a miscegenation of races, each region has a greater number of some type of race (MORAES; OLIVEIRA; COSTA, 2014).

With regard to marital status, more than half of the sample was single (56.25%), as in the study by Galvao et al. (2015), in which the percentage of single people was 73.3%.

Over the years, HIV/AIDS infection has taken on a characteristic of impoverishment related to the increase in the number of cases among people with low socioeconomic status: income less than or equal to one minimum wage and low schooling (MORAES; OLIVEIRA; COSTA, 2014).

The most frequent schooling levels were incomplete elementary school (43.75%) and complete elementary school (21.88%), corroborating results found in other studies with PLWHA such as those by Galvao et al. (2015), Camargo et al. (2014), Kroll et al. (2012) and Romancini et al. (2012) where 73.3%, 39.3%, 50.4% and 73.8% of their samples, respectively, had only completed elementary school.

There was a predominance of employed people (75%) corroborating the study by Galvao et al. (2015) in which the percentage was 66.6% and diverging from the study by Calvetti et al. (2014) in which there was a predominance of unemployed people (57.1%).

Regarding the economic conditions of the individuals, it was observed that, in general, they had an income of one minimum wage or less, a result that is in line with those of Moraes, Oliveira and Costa (2014) and Galvao et al. (2015) in which the frequency of individuals with the same income was 61.1% and 62.2%, respectively.

Camargo et al. (2014) in a study of 154 people living with HIV/AIDS and undergoing antiretroviral treatment reported that the participants reported that they used to use alcohol previously and 22.7% reported using it now; 25.3% used marijuana and 12.3% still do; 20.1% used cocaine and 1.3% use it now; 10.4% have used crack and 2.6% still use it. In line with this, Félix and Ceolim (2012) also had a sample in which the majority of individuals said they did not use alcohol (78.3%), cigarettes (73.3%) or drugs (98.3%). In this study, in addition to the majority having already consumed alcohol (87.5%) and used cigarettes (65.63%), 53.57% still consume alcohol and 47.62% say they continue to smoke.

Another approach to this issue comes from Fukumoto et al. (2013) who found smoking, alcoholism and other substance abuse in patients starting ART in 62.1% of the 58 patients who took part in the study, in addition to other comorbidities that also included depression.

In line with the study by Kroll et al. (2012), the majority of the individuals in this study's sample were also sedentary (75%). However, this differs, for example, from the study by Segatto et al. (2011) in which just under half of the individuals (45.2%)

were sedentary and also observed that there is an association between higher levels of physical activity and a lower incidence of lipodystrophy, where active individuals are 79% less likely to develop lipodystrophy when compared to sedentary individuals.

According to the BMI parameters proposed by ABESO (2009), 56.25% of the sample in this study had a normal weight. Similar findings can be found in the studies by Leite, Papa and Valentini (2011), Diehl et al. (2008) and Kroll et al. (2012), in which most of the individuals were also of normal weight (55%, 61% and 52.2%, respectively).

The findings of Diehl et al. (2008) in a study of 180 PLWHA suggest that 57% of patients had some change in their body shape after being diagnosed with HIV, and lipodystrophy was detected in 61% of patients who had been infected with HIV for six years and in 33% of those who had been infected for less than six years, and was more common in patients who had been infected with AIDS for eight years or more (74%). In line with these findings, more than 80% of the individuals in this study noticed some kind of change in their body.

With regard to self-assessment of appearance, 87.50% gave their appearance a score higher than 5, which differs from the study by Leite, Papa and Valentini (2011) where the majority of individuals were dissatisfied with their current physical shape (75%). Furthermore, after analysis, the authors observed that dissatisfied individuals had a higher proportion of complaints relating to depression, overweight and problems linked to treatment adherence, with individuals dissatisfied with their body image being 4.69 times more likely to be less adherent to antiretroviral treatment. They also suggest that satisfaction with body image is an important aspect to be explored in terms of adherence to treatment, mainly because it has the potential to be modified through interventions aimed at reducing body dissatisfaction and boosting self-esteem.

With regard to the presence of TMD in the PLWHA who took part in the study, only mild dysfunction was noted in most of them (53.13%). Other studies with other populations have also found only signs of mild dysfunction among the subjects and most of them were female (CAMACHO et al., 2014; OLIVEIRA et al., 2006).

Camacho et al. (2014) had a sample of 200 elderly people of both genders and observed the presence of TMD in 61% of the sample. Of these, 43.5% were considered mild, 13% moderate and 4.5% severe. When he associated this with gender, he found that 72.4% of women and 41.1% of men had some symptom of dysfunction and related the severity of TMD to the female gender.

Also in the study by Oliveira et al. (2006) with 2396 university students, the rate of individuals classified with mild TMD was significantly higher than those with other severity categories. Women presented some level of TMD at a higher frequency than men, but no significant difference for the same degree of severity between the sexes was observed.

Oliveira, Bevilaqua-Grossi and Dias (2008) studied the presence of TMD symptoms and university students and concluded that in different regions different levels of TMD can be found in university students and that the northeast and south regions are more likely to find university students with signs and symptoms of TMD than the others.

Donnarumma et al. (2010) carried out a retrospective study of 125 medical records of individuals who had undergone or were still undergoing treatment at a dental clinic and found that there was a predominance of women, with an average age of 35, with employment and greater complaints of pain in the TMJ region and clicking.

In this study, after applying the BDI, 21.88% of the subjects had no depression, 40.63% had mild depression, 28.13% had moderate depression and only 9.38% had severe depression. Silveira et al. (2012), in their study of 230 patients being treated at the SAE in Pelotas, found a prevalence of depressive symptoms of around 32%, with 14% having mild depression, 14% moderate depression and 4% severe depression, and associated the presence of depressive symptoms with gender, age, schooling, income, employment, social benefits and treatment regimen.

With regard to the association between lipodystrophy and the presence of TMD,

Fisher's test showed that there was no statistical association between the variables (p>0.05). And, as far as we know, no other study *has* tried to verify the association between these two variables.

We were also unable to observe a significant association between lipodystrophy and the presence of depression (p>0.05), although some authors have shown that the process of HIV infection, treatment, the implications of this process in the lives of these people, the adverse effects of treatment (SLHIV) and the low socioeconomic status of the majority of these individuals as risk factors for depression and low adherence to ART (GALVÂO et al., 2015; CAMARGO et al., 2014; MORAES; OLIVEIRA; COSTA, 2014; FUKUMOTO et al., 2013; KROLL et al., 2012; LEITE; PAPA; VALENTINI, 2011; SEGATTO et al., 2011; DIEHL et al., 2008).

However, an association between TMD and depression in people living with HIV/AIDS was observed (p=0.001), i.e. individuals with depression are more likely to develop TMD. These findings are in line with the literature.

Fernandes et al. (2013) in a sample of 224 individuals who sought care at a university clinic complaining of orofacial pain or for routine care, observed that 27.7% of the participants did not have TMD or it was not painful and 72.3% had chronic painful TMD. With regard to levels of depression, the presence of painful TMD and reports of tinnitus significantly increased the likelihood of moderate and severe levels of depression.

Similarly, Soares et al. (2012) selected a sample of 73 individuals aged between 18 and 62 years. At the end of the study, they observed that females were the most prevalent among patients with chronic TMD symptoms, that the most significant association was between the intensity of muscle symptoms and psychological impairment and that the continuation of TMD signs and symptoms for a prolonged period can lead to psychological manifestations.

The study was limited by the size of the sample, given that many of the research subjects did not want to be identified by people other than those in the SAE itself and by the refusal of many of the subjects who agreed to be approached by the researcher, a situation which resulted in a reduced number of subjects in the sample. A larger sample could have resulted in more significant results in the characterization and association of these variables. In addition, it was observed that some individuals probably answered some questions with the answers they thought were the most appropriate and not the true ones.

6. Conclusion

During the study, it was found that most of the participants were brown, had incomplete primary education, were single, had an income of less than or equal to one minimum wage, did not currently smoke, drank and did not exercise.

With regard to lipodystrophy, the majority had a normal weight, but noticed some kind of change in their body, whether in the face, arms, neck, breasts, waist, buttocks or thighs, and gave a score above 5 for their overall appearance. With regard to TMD, most had mild dysfunction and a few had severe dysfunction. With regard to the presence of depression, the majority showed signs of mild depression.

At the end of this study, it can be seen that there was no association between lipodystrophy and TMD and between lipodystrophy and depression, but there was a significant association between TMD and depression among PLWHA, where individuals with depression are more likely to develop TMD and these two variables seem to be proportionally related, i.e. the higher the level of depression, the greater the risk of TMD.

We also realized the need for interventions in this population, whether for prevention, promotion or health recovery, due to their risk situation and the characteristics found during the study. In this context, the role of nurses is of great importance in health education actions and in detecting signs and symptoms of depression and TMD in PLWHA, providing them with a better quality of life.

Although the study did not show a significant association between lipodystrophy, TMD and depression, the findings of this study may contribute to a better understanding of these phenomena in the lives of PLWHA and help develop intervention strategies with this population.

However, these results are not conclusive due to the limitations found in this study, such as the relatively small sample, which is likely to be a cross-sectional model, and non-probabilistic accidental sampling. Furthermore, other studies with a larger sample, different instruments and/or more variables related to lipodystrophy, TMD and depression are needed to corroborate these results.

7. REFERENCES

ANJOS, E.M.; PFRIMER, K; MACHADO, A. A; CUNHA, SFC C; SALOMÂO, R. G; MONTEIRO, JP Nutritional and metabolic status of HIV-positive patients with lipodystrophy during one year of follow-up. **Clinics** , Sao Paulo, v. 66, n. 3, p. 407-410, 2011. Available at: < http://www.scielo.br/scielo.php?script=sci_arttext&pid=S1807-59322011000300007&lng=en&nrm=iso >. Access em: 06 Jun. 2015.

ARMENTANO, TC; SILVA, A. R.; FERRARI, L. V; MATTHEUS, N. G; MELLO, R. The lipodystrophy in patients living with HIV / AIDS. **Revista de Pesquisa: Cuidado é Fundamental Online** , v. 5, n. 5, p. 173-181, Nov, 2013. Available at: <http://www.seer.unirio.br/index.php/cuidadofundamental/article   /view/1750>   . Access em: 06 Jun. 2015.

ASSOCIAÇÂO BRASILEIRA PARA O ESTUDO DA OBESIDADE E DA METABÒLICA SÌNDROME (ABESO). Diretrizes Brasileiras de Obesidade. 2009/2010. 3 ed. Itapevi, SP: AC Farmacêutica, 2009.

BONJARDIM, L. R.; GAVIÂO, MB D; PEREIRA, L.J.; CASTELO, P. M.; GARCIA, RCMR Signs and symptoms of temporomandibular disorders in adolescents . **Braz Oral Res** . Sao Paulo, v. 19, n. 2, p. 93-98, June, 2005. Available at:<   http://www.scielo.br/scielo.php?script=sci_arttext&pid=S1806-83242005000200004&Ing=en&nrm=iso >. Access em: 24 Apr. 2015.

BONOLO, P.F.; CECCATO, MG B; ROCHA, G.M .; ACÙRCIO, F. A; CAMPOS, L. N.; GUIMARÂES, MDC Gender differences in non-adherence among Brazilian patients initiating antiretroviral therapy. **Clinics,** Sao Paulo, v. 68, n. 5, p. 612 620, May, 2013. Available: < http://www.scielo.br/scielo.php?script=sci_arttext&pid=S1807-59322013000500612&lng=en&nrm= iso >. Access em: 01 Jun. 2015.

BÓSIO, JA A paradigm of relationship between occlusion, Orthodontics and temporal-mandibular dysfunction . **R Dental Press Orthodontic Orthopedic Facial**

. Maringà, v. 9, n. 6, p. 84-89, Nov/Dez, 2004. Available at: < http://www.scielo.br/pdf/dpress/v9n6/a12v9n6.pdf >. Access em: 24 Apr. 2015.

CALIXTRE, L. B; GRÜNINGER, BL S; CHAVES, T. C; OLIVEIRA, AB Is there an association between anxiety/depression and temporomandibular disorders in college students? **J Appl Oral Sci** ., v. 22, n. 1, p. 15-21, 2014. Available at: <http://dx.doi.org/10.1590/1678-775720130054> . Access em: 24 Apr. 2015.

CALVETTI, P. Ü; GIOVELLI, GR M; GAUER, GJ C; MORAES, JFD Psychosocial factors associated with adherence to treatment and quality of life in people living with HIV/AIDS in Brazil. **J. Bras. Psychiatrist** Rio de Janeiro, v. 63, n.

1, p. 8-15, Mar. 2014. Available at:

<   http://www.scielo.br/scielo.php?script=sci_arttext&pid=S0047-20852014000100008&lng=en&nrm=iso >. Access em: 01 Jun. 2015.

CAMACHO, JGD D; OLTRAMARI-NAVARRO, PV P; NAVARRO, R. L; CONTI, ACC F; CONTI, MR A; MARCHIORI, LL M; FERNANDES, KBP Signs and symptoms of Temporomandibular Disorders in the elderly. **CoDAS.** Sao Paulo, v. 26, n. 1, p. 76-80, Feb, 2014. Available at:

<   http://www.scielo.br/scielo.php?script=sci_arttext&pid=S2317-17822014000100076&lng=en&nrm=iso >. Access em: 17 May. 2015.

CAMARGO, B. V; BOUSFIELD, AB S; GIACOMOZZI, A. I; KOELZER, LP Representaçôes sociais e adesao ao tratamento antirretroviral. **LIBERABIT** : Lima (Perù), v. 20, n. 2, p. 229-238, 2014. Available at: http://revistaliberabit.com/es/revistas/liberabit20_2/4_vizeu.pdf. Access em: 06 Jun. 2015.

CAMARGO, L.A.; CAPITAO, C. G; FILIPE, EMV Mental health , familiar support e adesao ao tratamento: associaçôes no contexto HIV/Aids. **Psycho-USF** . Itatiba, v. 19, n. 2, p. 221-232, August, 2014. Available at:

<   http://www.scielo.br/scielo.php?script=sci_arttext&pid=S1413-82712014000200005&lng=en&nrm=iso >. Access em: 01 Jun. 2015.

CARMO FILHO, A et al. Factors associated with a diagnosis of major depression among HIV-infected elderly patients. **Revista da Sociedade Brasileira de Medicina Tropical** . v. 46, n. 3, p. 352-354, May-Jun. 2013.

CECCATO, MG B; BONOLO, P.F.; SOUZA NETO, A, I; ARAÙJO, F. S; FREITAS, MIF Antiretroviral therapy-associated dyslipidemia in patients from a reference center in Brazil. **Braz J Med Biol Res** . Ribeirao Preto, v. 44, n. 11, p. 1177-1183, Nov, 2011. Available at:

< http://www.scielo.br/scielo.php?script=sci_arttext&pid=S0100-879X2011001100015&lng=en&nrm=iso >. Access em: 01 Jun. 2015.

CHAVES, T. C; OLIVEIRA, A.S.; GROSSI, DB Principais instruments para avaliaçao da disfunçao temporomandibular, part I: indices e questionàrios; a contribution to clinical practice and research. **Physiotherapist. Fish** . Sao Paulo, v. 15, n. 1, p. 92-100, 2008. Available at:

< http://www.scielo.br/scielo.php?script=sci_arttext&pid=S1809-29502008000100015&lng=en&nrm=iso >. Accessed: May 19, 2015.

CORREIA, LM F; HUMMING, W; ADAMOWICZ, T; ALMEIDA, DB Importance of evaluating the presence of temporomandibular disorders in chronic pain patients. **Rev Dor** . Sao Paulo, v. 15, n. 1, p. 6-8, Jan/Mar, 2014. Available at: < http://www.scielo.br/pdf/rdor/v15n1/1806-0013-rdor-15 -01-0006.pdf >. Access em: 24 Apr. 2015.

DALL' ANTONIA, M; OLIVEIRA NETTO, R. M; SANCHES, M. L;

GUIMARÂES, AS Myofascial back muscular pain from mastigaçao is botulinum toxin . **rev. dor** , Sao Paulo, v. 14, n. 1, p. 52-57, Mar, 2013. Available: < http://www.scielo.br/scielo.php?script=sci_arttext&pid=S1806-00132013000100013&lng=en&nrm = iso >. Access em: 17 May. 2015.

DIEHL, L. A.; DIAS, J. R.; PAES, AC S; THOMAZINI, M. C; GARCIA, L. R.; KINAGAWA, E; WIECHMANN, S. L; CARRILHO, AJF The prevalence of HIV-associated lipodystrophy in Brazilian outpatients: relationship with metabolic syndrome and cardiovascular risk factors. **Arq Bras Endocrinol Metab** , Sao Paulo, v. 52, n. 4, p. 658-667, Jun, 2008. Available at: < http://www.scielo.br/scielo.php?script=sci_arttext&pid=S0004-27302008000400012&lng=en&nrm=iso >. Access em: 06 Jun. 2015.

DOMINGOS, H; CUNHA, R. V; PANIAGO, AM M; SOUZA, A.S.; RODRIGUES, R. L; DOMINGOS, JA Rosuvastatin e ciprofibrato no tratamento da dyslipidemia em pacientes com HIV. **Arch. Arm. Cardiol** . Sao Paulo, v. 99, n. 5, p. 997-1007, Nov, 2012. Available at:

< http://www.scielo.br/scielo.php?script=sci_arttext&pid=S0066-782X2012001400005&lng=en&nrm=iso >. Access em: 01 Jun. 2015.

DONNARUMMA, MD C; MUZILLI, C. A; FERREIRA, C; NEMR, K. Temporomandibular disorders : symptoms, symptoms and multidisciplinary approach. **rev. WHAT I DO** . Sao Paulo, v. 12, n. 5, p. 788-794, Out, 2010.

Available at: < http://www.scielo.br/scielo.php?script=sci_arttext&pid=S1516-18462010000500010&lng=en&nrm=iso >. Accessed: May 17, 2015.

DUTRA, CD T; LIBONATI, RMF Metabolic and nutritional approach to lipodystrophy em uso to antiretroviral therapy. **rev. Nutrition** Campinas, v. 21, n. 4, p. 439-446, August, 2008. Available at:

< http://www.scielo.br/scielo.php?script=sci_arttext&pid=S1415-52732008000400008&lng=en&nrm=iso >. Access em: 06 Jun. 2015.

EIRA, M; BENSENOR, I.M.; DOREA, E. L; CUNHA, R. S.; MILL, J.G.; LOTUFO, P. A. Highly *effective* antiretroviral therapy para infecçao pelo virus da immunodeficiência humana aumenta a stiffez aórtica. **Arch. Arm. Cardiol** . Sao Paulo, v. 99, n. 6, p. 1100-1107, Dec, 2012. Available at: < http://www.scielo.br/scielo.php?script=sci_arttext&pid=S0066-782X2012001500005&lng=en&nrm=iso >. Access em: 01 Jun. 2015.

FELIX, G; CEOLIM, MF A profile of a woman with HIV/AIDS is her addiction to antiretroviral therapy. **rev. Esc. Sick** . **USP** , Sao Paulo, v. 46, n. 4, p. 884 891, Aug,

2012. Available : < http://www.scielo.br/scielo.php?script=sci_arttext&pid=S0080-62342012000400015&lng=en&nrm= iso >. Access em: 01 Jun. 2015.

FERNANDES, G. et al. Painful temporomandibular disorders, self-reported tinnitus, and depression are highly associated. **Arch. Neuro-Psychiatr.** , Sao Paulo, v. 71, n. 12, p. 943-947, Dec. 2013. Available at: < http://www.scielo.br/scielo.php?script=sci_arttext&pid=S0004-282X2013001300943&lng=en&nrm=iso >. Access em: 9 Nov. 2015.

FONSECA, D. M et al. Diagnosis by anamnesis of craniomandibular dysfunction. **Rev. Gaucha Odontol** . v. 42, p. 23-8. 1994.

FUKUMOTO, AEC G; OLIVEIRA, C. C; TASCA, K. I; SOUZA, LR Evolution of patients with AIDS after cART: clinical and laboratory evolution of patients with AIDS after 48 weeks of antiretroviral treatment. **rev. Inst. Med. trope S. Paulo** , Sao Paulo, v. 55, n. 4, p. 267-273, Aug, 2013. Available at: < http://www.scielo.br/scielo.php?script=sci_arttext&pid=S0036-46652013000400267&lng =en&nrm=iso >. Access em: 01 Jun. 2015.

GALVAO, MT G; SOARES, L.L.; PEDROSA, S. C; FIUZA, ML T; LEMOS, LA Qualidade de vida e adesao à medicaçao antirretroviral em pessoas com

HIV. **Acta Paul. Sick** Sao Paulo, v. 28, n. 1, p. 48-53, Feb, 2015. Available at: < http://www.scielo.br/scielo.php?script=sci_arttext&pid=S0103-21002015000100048&lng=en&nrm=iso >. Access em: 01 Jun. 2015.

GODOI, ETA M; BRANDT, C. T; GODOI, JTA M; LACERDA, H.R.; ALBUQUERQUE, VM G; ZIRPOLI, J. C; GODOI, JTA M; SARTESCHI, C. The effect of antiretroviral therapy is two levels of viral load no complexo médio-intimal e no index tornozelo-braço em pacientes infectedos pelo HIV. **J. Vasc. Arm.** Porto Alegre, v. 11, n. 2, p. 123-131, Jun, 2012. Available at: < http://www.scielo.br/scielo.php?script=sci_arttext&pid=S1677-54492012000200009&lng=en&nrm=iso >. Access em: 01 Jun. 2015.

GONÇALVES, M. C; FLORENCIO, L. L; CHAVES, T. C; SPECIALI, J. G;

BIGAL, M. E; BEVILAQUA-GROSSI, D. Do women with migraine have higher prevalence of temporomandibular disorders? **Braz J Phys Ther** . v. 17, n. 1, p. 64-68. Jan-Feb, 2013. Available at: < http://dx.doi.org/10.1590/ S1413-35552012005000054 >. Access em: 23 Apr. 2015.

GUIMARÂES, PM et al. Suicide risk and alcohol and drug abuse in outpatients with HIV infection and Chagas disease. **Revista Brasileira de Psiquiatria** . Cities. v. 36, p. 131-137. 2014. Available at:

http://www.scielo.br/scielo.php?script=sci_arttext&pid=S1516-44462014000200131&lng=en&nrm=iso. Accessed: 01 Nov 2015.

HELKIMO, M. Studies on function and dysfunction of the masticatory system, II: index for anamnestic and clinical dysfunction and occlusal state. **Sven Tandlak Tidskr** . v. 67, n. 2, p. 101-21. 1974.

JANUZZI, E; ALVES, BM F; GROSSMANN, E; LEITE, FM G; VIEIRA, PS R; FLECHA, OD Occlusion and temporomandibular disorders: a critical analysis of the literature. **Rev Dor** . Sao Paulo, v. 11, n. 4, pp. 329-333. Out-dez, 2010. Available at: <http://files.bvs.br/upload/S/1806-0013/2010/v11n4/a1657.pdf> . Acesso em: Apr. 23 2015.

JUSTINA, LBD **The prevalence of lipodystrophy and associated factors in people living with HIV** . Tubarao, 2013. 85f. Dissertaçao (Master's Degree) - Universidade do Sul de Santa Catarina. Available to:

< http://www.uniedu.sed.sc.gov.br/wp-content/uploads/2014/04/Lunara-Basqueroto-Della-Justina.pdf >.

KROLL, A. F; SPRINZ, E. LEAL, S. C; LABRÊA, M. G; SETÙBAL, S. Prevalence of obesity and cardiovascular risk in patients with HIV/AIDS in Porto Alegre, Brazil. **Arq Bras Endocrinol Metab** , Sao Paulo, v. 56, n. 2, p. 137-141, Mar, 2012.

Available at: < http://www.scielo.br/scielo.php?script=sci_arttext&pid=S0004-27302012000200007&lng=en&nrm=iso >. Access em: 01 Jun. 2015.

LEITE, LH M; POPE, A; VALENTINI, RC Dissatisfaction with body image is frequent in antiretroviral therapy among individuals with HIV/AIDS. **rev.**

Nutrition , Campinas, v. 24, n. 6, p. 873-882, Dec, 2011. Available : < http://www.scielo.br/scielo.php?script=sci_arttext&pid=S1415-52732011000600008&lng=en&nrm=iso >. Access em: 01 Jun. 2015.

LEITE, R. A; RODRIGUES, J. F.; SAKIMA, M. T; SAKIMA, T. Relationship between temporomandibular disorders and orthodontic treatment: A literature review. **Dental Press J Orthod** . v. 18, n. 1, p. 150-157, Jan/Feb, 2013. Available at: < http://www.scielo.br/pdf/dpjo/v18n1/27.pdf >. Access em: 23 Apr. 2015.

MACHADO, I. M et al. Relaçao dos Sintomas Otológicos nas Dysfunçôes Temporomandibulares . **Arch. International Otolaryngology. / Intl. Arch. Otorhinolaryngol.** São Paulo. v. 14, n. 3, p. 274 - 279, Jul/Ago/Setembro - 2010. Available at: <http://www.arquivosdeorl.org.br/conteudo/pdfForl/14-03-02.pdf> . Access em: 24 Apr. 2015.

MALUF, TPG **Evaluation of symptoms of depression and anxiety in a sample of family members of drug users who frequent familiar grupos de orientação em um serviço asistencial para dependentes quimicos** . Sao Paulo, 2002. 59 pp. Theses (Mestrado) - Escola Paulista de Medicina, Universidade Federal de Sao Paulo.

MAYORAL, V. A; ESPINOSA, I. A; MONTIEL, A. J. Association between signs and symptoms of temporomandibular disorders and pregnancy (case control study). **Acta Odontol. I'm Latino** . v. 26, n. 1, p. 3-7. Available at: <http://actaodontologicalat.com/archivo/v26n1/01.pdf> . Access em: 23 Apr. 2015.

MAZZETTO, M. O; RODRIGUES, C. A; MAGRI, L. V; MELCHIOR, M. O; PAIVA, G. Severity of TMD Related to Age, Sex and Electromyographic Analysis. **Brazilian Dental Journal** . v. 25, n. 1, p. 54-58. 2014. Available at: <http://dx.doi.org/10.1590/0103-6440201302310> . Access em: 24 Apr. 2015.

MORAES, DC A; OLIVEIRA, R. C; COSTA, SFG Adesao de homens vivendo com HIV/Aids ao tratamento antirretroviral. **Esc. Anna Nery** , Rio de Janeiro, v. 18, n. 4,

p.   676-681,   Dec.   2014.   Available   at: <
http://www.scielo.br/scielo.php?script=sci_arttext&pid=S1414-
81452014000400676&lng=en&nrm=iso >. Access em: 01 Jun. 2015.

MORENO, BG D; MALUF, S.A.; MARQUES, A. P; CRIVELLO-JUNIOR, O.
Clinical evaluation and quality of life of individuals with temporomandibular
dysfunction. **rev. Arm. Physiotherapist** . Sao Carlos, v. 13, n. 3, p. 210-214, Jun,
2009. Available at: < http://www.scielo.br/scielo.php?script=sci_arttext&pid=S1413-
35552009000300004&lng=en&nrm=iso >. Access em: 17 May. 2015.

OLIVEIRA, A.S.; DIAS, E.M.; CONTATO, R. G; BERZIN, F. Prevalence study of
signs and symptoms of temporomandibular disorder in Brazilian college students.

Braz Oral Res . São Paulo, v. 20, n. 1, p. 3-7, Mar. 2006. Available at: <
http://www.scielo.br/scielo.php?script=sci_arttext&pid=S1806-
83242006000100002&Ing=en&nrm=iso >. Access em: 24 Apr. 2015.

OLIVEIRA, A.S.; BEVILAQUA-GROSSI, D; DIAS, EM Sinais e sintomas da
disfunçâo temporomandibular nas diferentes regiôes brasileiras. **Fisioterapia e
Pesquisa** , Sâo Paulo, v. 15, n. 4, p.392-397, out/dec. 2008. Available at: <
www.scielo.br/pdf/fp/v15n4/13.pdf >. Access em: 24 Apr. 2015.

OLIVEIRA, FBM **Avaliaçâo da qualidade de vida em pessoas vivendo com
HIV/AIDS** . Teresina, 2014. 102f. Dissertação (Master's Degree) - Universidade
Federal do Piaui.

OLIVEIRA, N.M.; FERREIRA, FA Y; YONAMINE, R. Y; CHEHTER, EZ
Antiretroviral drugs and acute pancreatitis in patients with HIV/AIDS: are there any
associations? Review the literature. **Einstein (Sao Paulo)** , Sao Paulo. v. 12, n. 1, p.
112-119, Mar. 2014. Available at:

<   http://www.scielo.br/scielo.php?script=sci_arttext&pid=S1679-
45082014000100022&lng=en&nrm=iso >. Access em: 01 Jun. 2015.

OLIVEIRA, OC A; OLIVEIRA, R. A; SOUZA, LR Impact of antiretroviral
treatment on the occurrence of macrocytosis in patients with HIV/AIDS in the

municipality of Maringà, Estado do Paranâ. **rev. Shock. Arm. Med. Too much** . Uberaba, v. 44, n. 1, p. 35-39, Feb, 2011. Available:

< http://www.scielo.br/scielo.php?script=sci_arttext&pid=S0037-86822011000100009&lng=en&nrm=iso >. Access em: 01 Jun. 2015.

ORTEGA, AO L; GUIMARÂES, AS Risk factors for temporomandibular dysfunction and orofacial pain in childhood and adolescence. **Rev Assoc Paul CiR Dent** . v. 67, n. 1, p. 14-17. 2013. Available at: < http://revodonto.bvsalud.org/pdf/apcd/v67n1/a02v67n1.pdf >. Access em: 23 Apr. 2015.

PADOIN, SM M; ZÜGE, S. S; ALDRIGHI, J.D.; PRIMEIRA, M.R.; SANTOS, EE P; PAULA, CC Mulheres do Sul Brasil em antiretroviral therapy: perfil eo cotidiano medicamentoso. **Epidemiol. Service Saùde** , Brasilia, v. 24, n. 1, p. 71 78, Mar, 2015. Available at:

< http://www.scielo.br/scielo.php?script=sci_arttext&pid=S2237-96222015000100071&lng=en&nrm=iso >. Access em: 01 Jun. 2015.

PASINATO, F; SOUZA, J. A; CORRÊA, EC R; SILVA, AMT Temporomandibular disorder and generalized joint hypermobility: application of diagnostic criteria. **Arm. J. Otorhinolaryngol** . Sao Paulo, v. 77, n. 4, p. 418 425, Aug. 2011. Available at:

< http://www.scielo.br/scielo.php?script=sci_arttext&pid=S1808-86942011000400003&lng=en&nrm=iso >. Access em: 17 May. 2015.

PEREIRA, G.S.; DUARTE, J.M.; VILELA, EM Evaluation of ocular symptoms in patients with temporo-mandibular dysfunction . **Arch. Arm. Ophthalmol.** Sao Paulo, v. 63, n. 4, p. 263-267, August, 2000. Available at:

< http://www.scielo.br/scielo.php?script=sci_arttext&pid=S0004-27492000000400004&lng=en&nrm=iso >. Access em: 17 May. 2015.

PIZOLATO, R. A; FERNANDES, FS F; GAVIÂO, MBD Anxiety/depression and orofacial myofacial disorders as factors associated with TMD in children. **Braz Oral Res** . Sao Paulo, v. 27, n. 2, p. 156-162, Abr. 2013. Available at:

< http://www.scielo.br/scielo.php?script=sci_arttext&pid=S1806-83242013000200156&lng=en&nrm=iso >. Access em: 23 Apr. 2015.

R Core Team. **A: A language and environment for statistical computing** . R Foundation for Statistical Computing. Vienna, Austria. (2015). Available at: http://www.R-project.org/. Accessed: 08 Nov 2015.

REIS, A. C; LENCASTRE, L; GUERRA, M.P.; REMOR, E. Relaçao entre sintomatologia psicopatológica, adesao ao tratamento e qualidade de vida na infecçao HIV e AIDS. **Psychol. Reflex. Crit.** Porto Alegre, v. 23, n. 3, p. 420-429. 2010.

Available at: < http://www.scielo.br/scielo.php?script=sci_arttext&pid=S0102-79722010000300002&lng=en&nrm=iso >. Access em: 01 Jun. 2015.

REIS, RK et al. Sintomas de depressao e qualidade de vida de pessoas vivendo com HIV/aids . **rev. Latin Am. We nurse** . v. 19, n. 4, t. 08, Jul-Aug. 2011.

Available to: http://www.revistas.usp.br/rlae/article/view/4390. Accessed : 01 Nov 2015.

ROMANCINI, JL H; GUARILHA, D; NARDO JR, N; HEROLD, P; PIMENTEL, GG A; PUPULIN, A. R. T. Levels of physical activity and metabolic alterations in pessoas vivendo com HIV/AIDS. **Rev Bras Med Esporte** , Sao Paulo, v. 18, n. 6, p. 356-360, Dec, 2012. Available at:

< http://www.scielo.br/scielo.php?script=sci_arttext&pid=S1517-86922012000600001&lng=en&nrm=iso >. Access em: 01 Jun. 2015.

ROSSI, SM G; MALUF, EC P; CARVALHO, D.S.; RIBEIRO, CE L;

BATTAGLIN, CRP Impacto da terapia antirretroviral conforme diferentes consensos de tratamento da Aids no Brasil. **Rev Panam Salud Publica** , Washington, v. 32, n. 2, Aug, 2012. Available at:

< http://www.scielosp.org/scielo.php?script=sci_arttext&pid=S1020-49892012000800005&lng=en&nrm=iso >. Access em: 06 Jun. 2015.

SANTOS, EC A; BERTOZ, F. A; PIGNATTA, LM B; ARANTES, FMA Clinical evaluation of signs and symptoms of temporomandibular dysfunction in children. **R Dental Press Orthodontic Orthopedic Facial** . Maringà, v. 11, n. 2, p. 29-34, Mar/Apr 2006. Available at:

< http://www.scielo.br/scielo.php?script=sci_arttext&pid=S1415-54192006000200005&lng=en&nrm=iso >. Access em: 24 Apr. 2015.

SEGATTO, AF M; FREITAS JUNIOR, I. F; SANTOS, V. R.; ALVES, KC P;

BARBOSA, D. A; PORTELINHA FILHO, A. M; MONTEIRO, HL Lipodystrophy in HIV/AIDS patients with different levels of physical activity while on antiretroviral therapy. **rev. Shock. Arm. Med. Trop** ., Uberaba, v. 44, n. 4, p. 420-424, August, 2011. Available at:< http://www.scielo.br/scielo.php?script=sci_arttext&pid=S003786822011000400004 &lng=en&nrm=iso >. Access em: 06 Jun. 2015.

SENA, M.F.; MESQUITA, KS F; SANTOS, FR R; SILVA, FWG P; SERRANO, KVD Prevalence of temporomandibular dysfunction in children and adolescents. **rev. paul pediatrician** Sao Paulo, v. 31, n. 4, pp. 538-545, Dec, 2013.

Available at: < http://www.scielo.br/scielo.php?script=sci_arttext&pid=S0103-05822013000400538&lng=en&nrm=iso >. Access em: 17 May. 2015.

SHARMA, S; GUPTA, D.S.; PAL, US; JUREL, SK Etiological factors of temporomandibular joint disorders. **Natl J Maxillofac Surg** . V. 2, p. 116-9. 2011.

SIGNORINI, DJH P; MONTEIRO, MC M; ANDRADE, MF C;

SIGNORINE, D. H; EYER-SILVA, WA What should we know about metabolic syndrome and lipodystrophy in AIDS?. **rev. Assoc. Med. Arms** . Sao Paulo, v. 58, n. 1, p. 70-75, Feb, 2012. Available to:

< http://www.scielo.br/scielo.php?script=sci_arttext&pid=S0104-42302012000100017&lng=en&nrm=iso >. Access em: 06 Jun. 2015.

SILVA, AC O; REIS, R. K; NOGUEIRA, J. A; GIR, E. Quality of life, clinical characteristics and treatment adherence of people living with HIV/AIDS. **rev.**

Latin Am. We nurse . Ribeirao Preto, v. 22, n. 6, p. 994-1000, Dec. 2014. Available at: < http://www.scielo.br/scielo.php?script=sci_arttext&pid=S0104-11692014000600994&lng=en&nrm=iso >. Access em: 01 Jun. 2015.

SILVA, G. A; TAKAHASHI, RF A busca pela assistance à saùde: reduzindo a vulnerabilidade ao doecimento entre os portatores do HIV. **rev. APS** , v. 11, n. 1, p. 29-41, Jan/Mar, 2008. Available at: <http://www.ufjf.br/nates/files/2009/12/029-041.pdf> . Access em: May 18. 2015.

SILVEIRA, MP T; GUTTIER, M. C; PINHEIRO, CA T; PEREIRA, TV S; CRUZEIRO, AL S; MOREIRA, LB Depressive symptoms in HIV-infected patients treated with highly active antiretroviral therapy. **rev. Arm. Psiquiatr.**, Sao Paulo, v. 34, n. 2, p. 162-167, Jun, 2012. Available at: < http://www.scielo.br/scielo.php?script=sci_arttext&pid=S1516-44462012000200008&lng= en&nrm=iso >. Access em: 01 Jun. 2015.

SOARES, FM G; COSTA, IMC Facial lipoatrophy associated with HIV/AIDS: do advento aos congementos atuais. **Year. Arm. Dermatol** . Rio de Janeiro, v. 86, n. 5, p. 843-864, Out, 2011. Available at:

< http://www.scielo.br/scielo.php?script=sci_arttext&pid=S0365-05962011000500001&lng=en&nrm=iso >. Access em: 06 Jun. 2015.

SOARES, FM G; COSTA, IMC Treatment of HIV-associated facial lipoatrophy: impact on infection progression assessed by viral load and CD4 count. **Year. Arm. Dermatol.** Rio de Janeiro, v. 88, n. 4, p. 570-577, Aug, 2013. Available at: < http://www.scielo.br/scielo.php?script=sci_arttext&pid=S0365-05962013000400570&lng=en&nrm= iso >. Access em: 06 Jun. 2015.

SOARES, T.V. et al . Correlaçao entre severidade da disordem temporomandibular e factori psicossociais em pacientes com chronic pain. **Odontol. Clin.-Scient.**

(Online) . Recife, v. 11, n. 3, set. 2012. Available at:

< http://revodonto.bvsalud.org/scielo.php?script=sci_arttext&pid=S1677-38882012000300005&lng=pt&nrm=iso >. Acesso em: 08 Nov. 2015.

TESCH, R.S.; URSI, WJ S; DENARDIN, OVP Epidemiological bases for analysis of more morphological occlusions as risk factors for temporomandibular disorders of articular origin. **R Dental Press Orthodontic Orthopedic Facial** . Maringà, v. 9, n. 5, p. 41-48, set/out. 2004. Available at: < http://www.scielo.br/scielo.php?script=sci_arttext&pid=S1415-54192004000500006&lng=en&nrm=iso >. Access em: 23 Apr. 2015.

TUFANO, C.S.; AMARAL, R. A; CARDOSO, LR D; MALBERGIER, A. The influence of depressive symptoms and substance use on adherence to antiretroviral therapy. A cross-sectional prevalence study. **Sao Paulo Med. J.** , Sao Paulo, 2015. Available at: < http://www.scielo.br/scielo.php?script=sci_arttext&pid=S1516-31802014005050010&lng=en&nrm=iso >. Accessed: 01 Jun 2015.

VALDÉS, M. S; ACOSTA, JE C; BRITO, I.M .; SARDINA, C. O. P; SARDINA, DP Factores de riesgo de la disfunción temporomandibular asociados al Test de Krogh Paulsen. **Rev Med Electron** . Matanzas, v. 32, n. 5. out. 2010. Available at: < http://scielo.sld.cu/scielo.php?script=sci_arttext&pid=S1684-18242010000500004&lng=es&nrm=iso >. Access em: 23 Apr. 2015.

VIANA, GM C; NASCIMENTO, MDS B; FERREIRA, A. M; RABELO, EM F; DINIZ NETO, J. A; GALVÂO, C. S; SANTOS, A. C; SANTOS JUNIOR, O. M; OLIVEIRA, RA S; BINDA JUNIOR, JR Evaluation of laboratory markers of progression of HIV disease to death **. rev. Shock. Arm. Med. Trop** ., Uberaba, v. 44, n. 6, p. 657-660, Dec. 2011. Available at:

< http://www.scielo.br/scielo.php?script=sci_arttext&pid=S0037-86822011000600001&lng=en&nrm=iso >. Access em: 01 Jun. 2015.

ZAVANELLI, A. C; ZUIM, PR J; BARBOZA, G.S.; JUSTI, MM Disfunçao temporomandibular na visao de professionales e acadêmicos de odontologia. **Studies of Psychology** . Campinas, v. 30, n. 4, p. 553-559, Dec. 2013. Available at: < http://www.scielo.br/scielo.php?script=sci_arttext&pid=S0103-166X2013000400008&lng=en&nrm=iso >. Access em: 24 Apr. 2015.

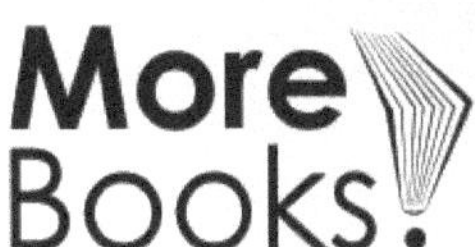

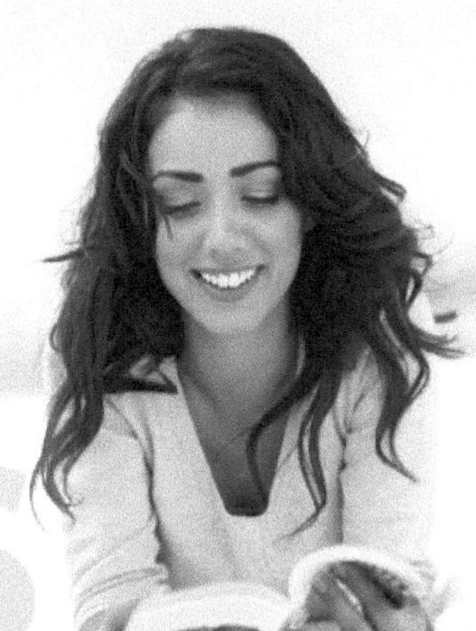

I want morebooks!

Buy your books fast and straightforward online - at one of world's fastest growing online book stores! Environmentally sound due to Print-on-Demand technologies.

Buy your books online at
www.morebooks.shop

Kaufen Sie Ihre Bücher schnell und unkompliziert online – auf einer der am schnellsten wachsenden Buchhandelsplattformen weltweit! Dank Print-On-Demand umwelt- und ressourcenschonend produziert.

Bücher schneller online kaufen
www.morebooks.shop

info@omniscriptum.com
www.omniscriptum.com

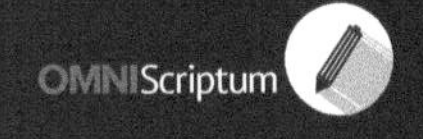

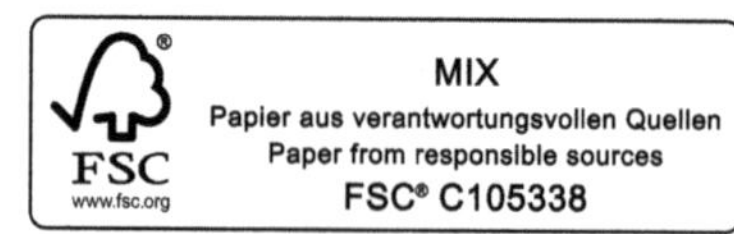

Printed by Books on Demand GmbH, Norderstedt / Germany